Pregnancy
Be Perfectly Pregnant

The ultimate guide to a Healthy, Happy pregnancy

By Linda Ledwidge

Note: the information in this book is true and complete to the best of my knowledge and understanding in this changing world.

The information and advice published in or made available through this book is not intended to replace the services of your physician. You should consult a physician in all matters relating your own health, and pregnancy, particularly in respect to any symptoms that may require diagnosis or medical attention.

The author makes no representations or warranties with respect to any information offered or provided in or through this book regarding treatment, action, or application of medication.

For my munchkins
Keri, Niki & PJ
My reason for Being
zoot, zoot, zoot
xcxcxc

Special thanks

~

With special thanks to my family and amazing circle of friends who always support me every step of the way.

Cover design - Marie Tillbert - you rock!

And last and most importantly,
Mum
For growing me, birthing me and nurturing me,
I love you xc

Pregnancy is not an illness.
It is a state of becoming...
2 becoming 3...or more!

~ Linda Ledwidge ~

Contents

The purpose of this book

Chapter 1 - We're Pregnant!

Chapter 2 - Being Perfectly Pregnant is natural.

Chapter 3 - How do you know that you are pregnant?

Chapter 4 –So...when are you due?

Chapter 5 - I´m going to be a Dad.... WOW!...OMG!

Chapter 6 – So, what do I need to know?

Chapter 7 – Myths exploded!

Chapter 8 - All about U-turns

Chapter 9 - So what's next?

Thank you

Resources

The purpose of this book

This book is a reminder that life is simple until we complicate it.
I want to thank you and congratulate you for purchasing
 "Pregnancy: Be Perfectly Pregnant
The ultimate guide to a Healthy, Happy pregnancy"

In 1988, I qualified as a midwife and over the last 29 years I am
fortunate enough to have grown, birthed, and raised 3 wonderful
children.
During almost 30 years providing antenatal, postnatal and birthing
advice I have connected to hundreds of parents now living all over the
world.
My eldest daughter is now growing her own Baby and I am going to
be a Grandma, Granny, Nan or whatever magical word my grandchild
decides to use to describe our relationship when the time comes.
I am passionate about helping prospective families to have the best
pregnancy and birthing experience possible for them no matter what.
Nothing you will read in this book is new, however, much of what you
will read has been forgotten over time and that has led to the high
incidence of "medical" births that we see today.
I am not advocating the demise of doctors or hospitals in pregnancy
and childbirth. I am simply exploring reasons why "nature´s miracle"
has become this thing to be feared.
Pregnancy is **not** an illness and yet it has become the norm to treat it
as such.
There is no reason that a woman cannot give birth in the "safety" of a
medical environment and have a wonderful experience.
How can we make that more of a reality in our society today?

*Eliminate the fear factor and you will
eliminate the majority of complications.
It really is all about how you feel!*

~ Linda Ledwidge ~

I have attempted, with this book, to bring the focus back to what we know to be true. Being pregnant and giving birth is one (three) of the most satisfying things I have done in my life. I have no regrets about any of it although, with the knowledge that I have now I know that I could have had a better experience.

My wish is that all women, men and Babies who experience the wondrous world of pregnancy and childbirth do so without fear.

Thanks again for purchasing this book,
I hope you enjoy it!

I would really appreciate if you would write a short review, after reading (or a long one).

We're Pregnant!

Chapter 1

We're Pregnant!

*A*nd yes, I do mean we. It takes two and whether you like it or believe it or not, this baby is connected to you both.
It's just how it is.

I´m coming........

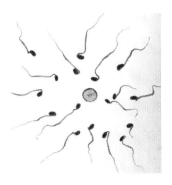

And so, it begins .....

That second when the test is positive is such a life - changing moment and the excitement builds.
All sorts of feelings emerge, like elation, joy, excitement...
then you tell other people, you start to think about what this means and you want information.

You want to know what's happening, what changes are taking place, what should you do, say, eat, think!!!
That's when it can get messy.

This is the time when everybody and their Auntie (as we say in Scotland) thinks that they have the right to verbally vomit all over You! and the "good" advice begins.
They mean well, they just don't realise the harm that they can cause.
We live in an information age and whilst that can be a wonderful thing, it can also cause a lot of confusion. You see everything you hear or read is from someone else´s perspective, this is what they have experienced, or heard, or read. This includes Mrs. Google, she who knows all!
That doesn't make it wrong, and it doesn't make it right, for you.

The aim of this book is to help you to find the calm in the storm.

*"It is the divine right of every woman to
Experience "nature´s miracle" :
Pregnancy and childbirth in her own unique way"*

~ Linda Ledwidge ~

Pregnancy is "nature´s miracle," it is the most natural thing in the world for a woman to become pregnant, grow and nurture her baby and then give birth.

*"It is every child´s divine right to enter this world
in his own unique way, when the time is right. "*

There are lots of books, websites and apps where you can find day by day / week by week/ month by month guides, where you can get every bit of information and knowledge on the changes, the complications, the expectations and the "right" things to do.

This book will not attempt to answer all your questions what it will do is guide you to the knowledge that is within you and help you to make some sense of the madness around you and recognise when something is "right" for you and your Baby.

Being Perfectly Pregnant is natural.

If being Perfectly Pregnant is natural, why do complications occur?

Chapter 2

Being Perfectly Pregnant is natural.

If being Perfectly Pregnant is natural, why do complications occur?

Quite simply because we get in the way of allowing nature to work.

The most important thing that you can do is to avoid ANYTHING that makes you feel "bad" or "uneasy."

That includes what you see, hear and read.

Does that seem too simple? The common answer is yes.

If you can grasp the truth of this you are well on the way to Being Perfectly Pregnant in your own way.

The human body has its own innate intelligence to maintain health, healing and growth. It will do whatever it takes, for as long as it can, to maintain that balance and survive.

This is never truer than in pregnancy because pregnancy is nature's own miracle.

Your body was made to conceive, grow and birth your Baby.

It knows exactly what to do, what it needs and when it's time to birth.

Your Baby's body knows exactly how to grow, what rate to develop at, what position is best for birth and when the time is right to come into this world.

Every cell in your body works in synergy and knows it´s purpose and the same is true for your Baby, from the first moment of fertilisation.

Let's look at how this all works.

BASIC NEEDS FOR LIFE

The fundamental needs for life are ...

OXYGENATION

Our breath is the life force that flows through us and this is what provides our 1st basic need - oxygen.

HYDRATION

The body is made up of 85% water; therefore to hydrate we need to make sure we drink plenty of good water.

RELAXATION

Relaxation allows flow. Without flow, there is tension which inhibits growth and healing.

BALANCE

The human body will always strive for balance, physical and chemical... Without balance, it cannot maintain health and development.

Life is about movement, growth and expansion.
Ease of movement or **flow** determines our state of being at any time.
Movement requires a connection to a power supply and ease of flow depends on what is in the way.

Our breath is our connection to our source, our power supply. Without breath, there is no life. Our breath connects the body, mind and spirit.

Breath is fundamental for life and during pregnancy, labour and birth our breathing signals to us what is going on and what is needed from us to help the process along.

In pregnancy and childbirth, your breathing is the **number 1** most important thing that you can focus on for a healthy Baby and a wonderful birthing experience.

You see it's ALL about FLOW!

When we have flow, we have ease, we have relaxation, and there is no interruption and no tension.

The way we are breathing is the first indicator that our subconscious mind gets when there is a problem .....

think about it.

When you are in pain. What do you do?

What happens when we have pain....

• WE HOLD OUR BREATH OR BREATHE IRREGULARLY

This leads to reduction of oxygen and blood flow to the tissues.

• THEN COMES THE TENSION

This causes tension in the body and increases the pain ....

obstruction or no flow...

• AND NO RELAXATION

Relaxation allows flow.

Without flow, there is tension and tension leads to pain or a problem!

• OFF BALANCE

....so now you are off balance and the pain gets worse.

As you can see, it all starts with a breath.

As soon as you focus on your breathing, you are sending a strong signal to your subconscious that you are safe. You may still feel the pain and struggle to breathe with ease, but when you get it under control the pain will instantly decrease. As soon as you get that breath flowing, your body starts to get back into balance:

- Oxygen flows to the tissues
- Blood flow is re-established
- The body then starts to release hormones to combat the pain and promote healing.

Were you aware that our body produces its own natural "painkillers" and anti-inflammatories?

It's the same with negative emotion like worry, anxiety, anger, and so on.... all causing tension and the first indication is a change in breathing.
When you are relaxed and happy your breath is flowing.

It follows then that when you are pregnant you want **flow** and the first step in getting there is to realise when there is interrupted or no flow, so that you can change it.
The way you feel gives you that sign and the first physical indication is a change in or holding your breath....no flow!

Notice how it works for you.
The next time you feel some tension or you are annoyed, become aware of how you are breathing and where you are holding tension in your body... Focus on taking nice calm, relaxed breaths and then notice what happens to the tension and your mood.
This is very simple and yet very powerful!

This is the awesome way that your body works when it is left to do what it does naturally!

How do you know that you are pregnant?

Chapter 3

How do you know that you are pregnant?

*Y*ou may have felt "something" and decided to take a pregnancy test or you may have had some other sign and / or symptom.

Here are some of the common signs that women have that signal pregnancy, the reason that it happens and some tips for how to cope.

Hormones are the body's chemical communication messengers and they control all bodily functions. Specific pregnancy hormones are so smart that they support your body's metamorphosis into whatever unique state is required for your baby's development, birth and nurturing.

Missed period

You may be a few days late or a couple of weeks late when you notice.

Ok, so here's why –

The egg is fertilised and your body is now preparing the uterus to receive it. Our little friends the chemical messengers have relayed the fact and therefore the lining of the womb grows instead of shedding.

Wow!

Tips
• Relax, this is a natural sign that things are progressing.

Blood Spotting

Sometimes you may get spots of blood accompanied with cramping, mood swings and headaches.
Can be mistaken for a light period as it will be around the time that menstruation is due. Can last for up to 2 days.

Ok, so here's why –

This is known as implantation bleeding.
If you have some blood spotting that indicates that the fertilised egg, now an embryo, has embedded in the womb. The spotting will be light, not a heavy bleed and brown or pink in colour.

Tips

- Rest if you feel tired.
- Drink plenty of water
- If you are concerned at all, get some advice. If not....
- Relax, this is a natural sign that things are progressing.

Tender breasts and nipples

This is one of the most common first signs of pregnancy - can have darkening of the areolas and veins may be pronounced.

Ok, so here's why –

Hormonal changes are:
- Preparing your milk ducts and storing fat to produce colostrum, which is Baby's first food.
- Increasing blood flow to the area
- The breasts may become very sensitive and can have significant visible changes.

Tips

- Wear a comfortable supporting bra. This will help prevent sagging and stretch marks.
- Let your partner know that he may not be able to touch

your breasts now, or show him how to touch you; this usually passes after the first 8 - 10 weeks.

- Relax, this is a natural sign that things are progressing.

May feel nausea with / without sickness

IF you have periods of nausea and / or sickness you will also have periods where you are hungry and want to eat - make sure you notice when this is and eat at these times.

Ok, so here's why –

In early pregnancy, there is tremendous growth and development happening. The two bodily processes that use the most energy are digestion and regeneration or growth. So, you see this is the body's way of letting you know that while it needs the nourishment and resources to grow your Baby; it also needs help with the process of digestion at the same time - *Very clever body!*

Tips
- Eat small amounts
- Eat food that is easily digested, like soups, juices, fresh food

• Cold food may help as hot food has more aroma and if your sense of smell is heightened this can make you more nauseous
• Eat slowly
• Drink plenty of water
• Ginger tea may help
• Relax, this is a natural sign that things are progressing.

Cravings or aversions to food or other things

Ok, so here's why –

Your body is talking to you, LISTEN! Craving certain foods can be a sign that your diet is deficient. Some examples are........*I know...laugh*, if you are craving these
- Coal / dirt / ice - this can indicate low iron
- Chocolate - low magnesium which is essential for growth
- Oily or fatty foods - low calcium
Aversions usually are because the body is using energy for growth and sends a signal that it does not want food right now.

Tips

- Recognise what the craving is and look for ways to incorporate it into your diet.
- When you feel an aversion to something avoid it! It's that simple!
- Relax, this is a natural sign that things are progressing.

Tiredness - more like exhaustion!

It's perfectly normal to feel this exhaustion in the early weeks.

Ok, so here's why –

In the first weeks of pregnancy your body is adapting to all the hormonal changes, finding the correct balance as well as preparing the uterus and laying the foundation for growing your Baby (formation of the placenta).

Your body is working hard to grow your Baby and it can do this optimally when you are out of the way, i.e. relaxed or preferably asleep! You see when you are fighting the tiredness or the nausea or the cravings or are just tense your Body has to work harder. So listen and take a nap and if you can´t nap take a few minutes to relax, take a breath and have a smile to yourself about the fact that you are an amazing human being, having an amazing experience.

Tips
- Make sure you are eating a nutritious diet that is rich in iron
- Eat little and often to maintain blood glucose levels.
- Get enough sleep and rest. Listen to your body.
- Exercise - a 10-minute walk every day will help you feel better as it will keep the blood and oxygen flowing.
- Practice breathing exercises to promote good oxygen flow.
- Relax, this is a natural sign that things are progressing.

Lots of peeing!

You will find that you have to pee much more often. This is the time to start with your pelvic floor exercises / AKA Kegels (see chapter 6)

AND CONTINUE FOR LIFE!

Ok, so here's why –

Hormonal changes and increased blood supply causes the

kidneys to work harder. Your womb is growing and this also puts pressure on the bladder.

Tips

- Drink plenty of water and go when you need to go, don't hold on to it!
- Caffeine can make you pee more so cut down on tea and coffee...oh and the Coca Cola!!
- Relax, this is a natural sign that things are progressing.

Heightened senses, especially smell

A heightened sense of smell can be one of the first signs of pregnancy. All senses are heightened to different degrees in all pregnant women.

Ok, so here's why –

Yes, it's the hormonal army again.

Blood flow is increased by as much as 50% in pregnancy. This means that there is a faster flow of blood moving through the brain and all senses are heightened.

This may be a protective mechanism as we are then more aware of any dangers to ourselves or our Baby. This will all settle down postnatally. There is a school of thought that says the increased sense of smell contributes to morning sickness.

Tips

- Stay away from what you don't like!
- If it tastes awful - don't eat it!
- If it smells awful - don't stay near it or smell it!
- If it feels strange - don't touch it!
- If it looks a bit gory- don't look at it!
- If it sounds horrific - don't listen!
- Relax, this is a natural sign that things are progressing.

This is a perfect sign that follows Be Perfectly Pregnant´s philosophy, your senses are telling you that this is not good for you, so do whatever it takes stay away or change it!

All that matters is how you feel!

Emotional see-saw

You are laughing one minute and the next the floodgates have opened up and the tears flow ...what's it all about?

Ok, so here's why –

This is often where the "don't worry it's her hormones" advice is dished out.

Yes, your body has hormones flying around perfecting a balancing act that any high wire artist would be proud of; however, that's what is supposed to be happening.

The reason for the emotional see-saw is not because your hormones are any different from anyone else, it's primarily because you are entering a new phase of your life and feel unprepared for it, no matter how prepared you thought you were.

Tips

• Be selfish! All that matters is how you feel. Your Baby's development depends on how you feel. Ask yourself whenever you do not feel good - do I want my Baby to feel like this? If so for how long?

• Talk to people, your partner, your doctor, midwife, mother, friend. Do not push away anything that you are concerned about.

• Rest when you need it. Take 10 minutes out, have a snack and boost your energy.

• Tell your partner if you are feeling insecure or worried.

Chances are they are feeling the same way. It's never as bad as you think! Left alone it can become huge.

- Relax, this is a natural sign that things are progressing.

Hot! Hot! Hot!

The menopause is not the sole cause of hot flashes. A woman's core temperature will be slightly higher during pregnancy.

Ok, so here's why –

Increased blood volume means that your blood vessels dilate and you have a greater blood flow to the skin surface, making you feel hot. This will all return to normal after the birth so make the most of being hot while you can!

Tips

- Drink! Drink! Drink! Plenty of water. Stay hydrated.
- Wear layers so that you can comfortably remove them.
- Carry a fan; it's a quick way to cool down.
- Relax, this is a natural sign that things are progressing.

Constipation and Bloating

Feeling bloated and constipated? - this too will pass!

Ok, so here's why –

Hormones! Hormones! Hormones! - yet again.

As I said earlier, digestion uses a lot of energy and so does growing your Baby. Baby needs nutrients as you do and some of the pregnancy hormones make the bowel a little sluggish to help with all of this.

You see, to make better use of the available energy, the food takes a little longer to digest, therefore the slowing of the bowel helps keep it around long enough for your Baby to get what he needs.

With your expanding uterus, the bowel will also have a little less room and this can also cause constipation.

Pregnancy supplements can also influence constipation. Take this into consideration and get your nutritional intake from whole foods as much as possible.

Tips
• Drink plenty of water - this helps with the absorption and

helps to keep the bowel moving. Warm water with lemon helps to stimulate the digestive tract.

• Eat small portions more often.

• Buy foods that will have a slightly higher fibre content than you are used to, such as fresh fruit, green veg and nuts.

• Choose foods that have a natural laxative effect - Aloe Vera, kiwi fruit, leafy green vegetables, prunes.

• Go for a stroll! Walking is one of the best exercises you can do and this will help activate the bowel.

• Relax, this is a natural sign that things are progressing.

You can see from all of this how amazing your body is, right. It knows you so well.

In fact, there is nobody more equipped to take care of you than you.

So ... when are you due?

Chapter 4

So ... when are you due?

*T*he first thing you will want to know and everyone you tell will ask is "when are you due"?

When you visit your doctor or midwife they will give you an EDD - estimated due date or "guesstimated" due date!

This is commonly worked out based on pregnancy duration of 40 weeks.

Everyone will tell you that a "normal" pregnancy lasts 40 weeks.

Your doctor will work out your EDD using the first day of your last menstrual period. So, using this method, as you can see, for at least the first 2 weeks of this 40-week pregnancy ...

YOU ARE NOT EVEN PREGNANT!

However, we like to have guidelines to help us prepare and that's a good thing to give you a focus.

A human pregnancy is approximately 39 - 41 weeks from the first day of the last menstrual period.

If you don´t know the date usually your obstetrician will use the scan to work it out, and of course they have universal guidelines that tell them how many weeks your Baby is based on measurements.

The important thing to remember is .....

Your body and your baby KNOW, no one else!

Babies develop at different rates and only your body and your Baby know when he is cooked.

Less than 5% of babies arrive on their EDD.

The reason I want to talk about this is that so many people get all hung up on the due date. Since time began babies have been born and the term of growth has varied in every pregnancy.

In our society, we like to "know" things.

No number of scans or calculations will tell you **exactly** what is happening and when your Baby is ready......however, your body and your Baby KNOW.

Let's imagine your scan to be a bit like looking through the oven door watching a cake bake....

- You can see the mixture you put in, all the ingredients mixed together
- You can see it rises slowly
- You watch as it changes colour and starts to look like a cake

- You have no idea how well it is cooked in the centre, so you follow the recipe temperature and timing
- There are times when no matter how well you follow the recipe your cake will need a little longer to cook

Scans today are wonderful. We can see our Baby in detail; however, remember that when he is fully cooked his timer will let you know in no uncertain terms!
Our society has decided that the gestation period (cooking time) of a human Baby is 40 weeks!

WE BUY INTO IT!

Your Baby will grow and develop at his own unique rate; there is no universal cooking time.

Relax and take it easy. You and your body have got this!

I´m going to be a Dad.... WOW! ...OMG!

Chapter 5

I´m going to be a Dad.... WOW! ...OMG!

Even when a pregnancy is planned most guys get an overwhelming feeling of panic when they hear the news... it's positive!

The thing about this is that they don´t think anyone will understand and they feel they have no one to talk to. Their concerns are generally about their partner's well-being, financial worries, or how good a parent they will be.

The first thing to understand is that you, as the father, have a strong connection to your Baby too. Yes, your partner has that physical connection as well as the emotional and energetic connection; however, your Baby is part of both of you. He shares your DNA and this is a real connection. I won't go into the physics of it all here because it would take too long and get too heavy, just know that it is so.

There is a 3 - way bond happening here and the way you feel and what you do affects your Baby as much as what your partner feels and does.

Why is this important?

Well because so many guys think that what they think, feel and do has no effect whatsoever on the baby, only on their partner. If you are feeling panic, tension, reacting badly to stress, while this will influence your partner, so you attempt to hide it (which you cannot), you really cannot hide it from your Baby. The direct connection that you have means that what you feel, your baby feels.

It's a 3 -way thing now!

The best way to handle this is to make sure that you communicate with each other and share concerns in a way that relieves any tension.

I usually explain it this way, guys' logic!

When you have engine problems with your car and it's kind of coughing and spluttering, what do you do?

Do you ignore it and hope it will go away? Or do you have a look under the bonnet (or get someone else to look)?

You see, you know that if there is something causing interference with the flow of the engine it will eventually result in a bigger issue, and usually cost you more.

It's the same with pregnancy. The issues being pregnant bring up for **both** of you can lead to some coughing and spluttering and if you do not look under the bonnet and resolve the issues it will lead to tension and then a bigger issue.

You see it's ALL about FLOW!

There is a lot of hype about hormonal changes, mood swings and how to deal with this. We hear this all through life, a woman's hormones are playing up when she's premenstrual, when she's menstrual, when she's pregnant, when she's in the menopause ..... give us a break!

Hormones are part of life, male and female.

Yes, there are a lot of hormones flying about and you may have to duck and dive a bit, however, they are all doing a great job and with some awareness and understanding of each other's feelings you can avoid any direct hits. Don't blame the hormones; it's all about how you feel...always!

Whenever there is tension there is some kind of fear or anxiety and if it's not addressed it WILL lead to a problem or issue, so just deal with it.

Talk to each other, if a subject is a bit delicate, find the right time and place. The best advice I can give you is not to ignore it and hope that it will go away.

It usually doesn´t.

So, what do I need to know?

Chapter 6

So, what do I need to know?

*T*here are obviously some essential changes that are unique to pregnancy.

• Your body releases hormones that make your bones, muscles and tissues more pliable.

This is important, as it allows the movement necessary for your Baby to grow and be birthed.

• Your body, from conception, prepares both you and your Baby for the development while pregnant and to nurture your Baby when he is born. This is seen predominantly in the changes in the breasts and production of colostrum and as the pregnancy progresses in the increased "bump" that begins to show.

• You have increased blood supply to your body giving it the strength it needs to nurture your developing Baby.

• Your baby will grow at his own rate. The systems of his body will develop, however, most of them do not actually mature until birth.

The reason for this is that he does not need them to actually function fully until birth.

Right from the start when you discover that you are pregnant there are 5 things that, if you focus on them throughout your pregnancy, will make such a difference to how you feel, how your Baby develops and how you cope with labour.

Breathing
Nutrition
Exercise
Relaxation
Connection

We could write a book on them all, so I am going to cover the basics here, which will make a significant difference, and if you want to find out more you can, by contacting me or researching further.

Breathing

Breathing is the most important thing in life and focused, conscious breathing can really make a difference to your pregnancy and labour.
That's because it maximises the amount of oxygen you and the Baby receive, and connects your mind, body, spirit and baby.

When this connection is broken, your body is out of balance and that creates fear and tension.

When we are frightened or in pain we hold our breath or it becomes shallow and rapid, and we tense all our muscles up; this sends a message to the brain that we are scared...

Fear =Tension = Pain / Problem

Breathing & relaxation exercises should be practiced throughout your pregnancy.

Simple breathing techniques

Close your eyes and focus on your breathing.
Notice the rhythm, in, pause and out, in, pause and out.
Your in- breath more or less matches your out-breath.
Now breathe deeply through your nose, breathe into your abdomen, fill the abdomen and then fill the lungs with air, expanding the lungs fully, pause and then breathe out through your mouth, making a sound as if you are shushing a Baby, slowly emptying the lungs and then the abdomen, expelling all the air in the lungs and taking all the toxins out of your body. Your out-breath should be at least 3 – 4 times longer than your in-breath.

Keep that rhythm going. Keep focused on the rhythm and keep your out-breath longer than your in-breath
It can help to practice breathing and relaxation techniques and strategies during pregnancy so that you can use them effectively in labour.

During labour and birth your breathing is your connection to what is happening with your Baby.
With each stage of labour and birth your breathing will change to aid the process if nothing gets in the way of that flow.
This is the basis for natural childbirth.

You see it's ALL about FLOW!

I recommend that you take the time to connect to your breath. Notice when it changes and why.
Building that connection will enable you and your Baby to experience a truly wonderful labour and birth.

Nutrition –
Healthy eating & supplements

Healthy eating is always important.

So, make sure your calories come from nutritious foods that will contribute to your baby's growth and development.

You know what foods you enjoy and what nourishes your body. Just because you are pregnant doesn't mean that you must change what you eat.

There are many myths about what you should avoid when pregnant (see Chapter 7 myths exploded) and so much of what you are led to believe really has no basis.

There has been lots of research done to provide information on this. A lot of what we read, hear and unfortunately are advised by well-meaning people, and professionals, is unfounded and the fact that it is repeated so often is what gives it substance.

Use logic and common sense and you will get there.

Maintain a well-balanced diet that incorporates
non - processed, whole foods including, if you enjoy them:

- Lean meats
- Fish
- Fruits
- Vegetables
- Whole-grain breads
- Dairy products
- Chocolate - YES chocolate!

By eating a healthy, balanced diet you're more likely to get
the nutrients you need.

You will need more of the essential nutrients (especially
magnesium, calcium, iron, and folic acid) than you did
before you became pregnant.

If you are taking prenatal vitamins it doesn't mean you can
eat a diet that's lacking in nutrients. It's important to
remember that you still need to eat well while pregnant.
Prenatal vitamins are meant to supplement your diet, and
aren't meant to be your only source of much-needed
nutrients.

Calcium

Calcium is more readily absorbed from:

- Almonds, Brazil nuts, hazelnuts
- Broccoli, curly kale, okra, spinach, watercress
- Dried apricot and figs
- Mackerel, oysters, pilchards, salmon, sardines
- Pulses, sesame seeds

Iron

Pregnant women need about 30 mg of iron every day.

Why?

Because iron is needed to make haemoglobin, the oxygen-carrying component of red blood cells. Red blood cells circulate throughout the body to deliver oxygen to all its cells.

Without enough iron, the body can't make enough red blood cells and the body's tissues and organs won't get the oxygen they need to function well.

So, it's especially important for pregnant women to get enough iron in their daily diets — for themselves and their growing babies.

Although the nutrient can be found in various kinds of foods, iron from meat sources is more easily absorbed by the body than iron found in plant foods.

Vitamin C helps the absorption of iron.

Iron-rich foods include:

- Red meat
- Dark poultry
- Salmon
- Eggs
- Tofu
- Enriched grains
- Dried beans and peas
- Dried fruits
- Dark leafy green vegetables

Magnesium:

Magnesium is essential for growth and regeneration of cells.

Magnesium rich foods include:

Almonds

Cashews

Brazil nuts

Seeds

Whole grains

Mackerel

Salmon

Leafy green vegetables especially spinach

Bananas

Exercise during pregnancy

Avoid lying flat on your back after 16 weeks, as it may make you feel faint.

Specific exercises to help the muscles include:

Stomach-strengthening exercises

As your bump gets bigger, you may find that the hollow in your lower back increases and this can give you backaches. These strengthen stomach (abdominal) muscles and ease backache, which can be a problem in pregnancy:

Cat Curl

• Start in a box position (on all fours) with knees under hips, hands under shoulders, with fingers facing forward and abdominals lifted to keep your back straight.

• Pull in your stomach muscles and raise your back up towards the ceiling, curling the trunk and allowing your head to relax gently forward. Don't let your elbows lock.

• Hold for a few seconds then slowly return to the box position

• **IMPORTANT!!!!** Take care not to hollow your back: it should always return to a straight/neutral position.

• Do this slowly and rhythmically 10 times, making your muscles work hard and moving your back carefully.

• Only move your back as far as you can without discomfort.

Pelvic tilt exercises

• Stand with your shoulders and bottom against a wall.
• Do not lock your knees.
• As you breathe in - Pull your tummy button towards your spine, so that your back flattens against the wall: hold for four seconds and release breathing out.
• Repeat up to 10 times.

Pelvic floor exercises

- YOU WILL DO THESE FOR LIFE!
(If you are smart)

Pelvic floor muscles are extremely stressed during pregnancy and when the baby is born. The pelvic floor consists of layers of muscles that stretch like a supportive hammock from the pubic bone (in front) to the end of the backbone (coccyx).

If your pelvic floor muscles are weak, you may find that you leak urine when you cough, sneeze or strain. This is quite common and you needn't feel embarrassed.

It's known as stress incontinence and it can continue after pregnancy. By performing pelvic floor exercises, you can strengthen the muscles. This helps to reduce or avoid stress incontinence after pregnancy. All pregnant women should do pelvic floor exercises, even if you're young and not suffering from stress incontinence now.

*********** *NOTE!!!!* ********
This also makes your sex life much more enjoyable for both of you!!!

How to do pelvic floor exercises:

DO THIS EXERCISE WITH AN EMPTY BLADDER
• Imagine there is a string coming out of your belly button and you are pulling on it. Start from there NOT from the back.
• So, you pull on the string and it tightens your abdomen.
• Tighten your urethra like when you want to stop peeing.
• Then slowly tighten your vagina as if you're gripping a tampon, and then your buttocks and your anus as if you're trying to stop your bowels moving.
• Do this exercise every time you go to the toilet **after** peeing, while washing your hands.
• Do it quickly, then do it slowly, holding the contractions for as long as you can before you relax: try to count to 10.

• As well as these exercises, practice tightening up the pelvic floor muscles before and during coughing and sneezing.

Remember: DO THIS EXERCISE WITH AN EMPTY BLADDER

Using a gym ball / pregnancy ball

Always sit with knees slightly more than hip width apart, feet flat on the floor, back straight and arms relaxed at your side.

1. Bounce up and down as you breathe slowly and consciously, this relaxes you and the baby. Connect to your body and your baby. Ask Baby how he feels, what he needs. Tell him you love him. See him in the womb perfect and growing, everything as it should be.

2. Move your pelvis clockwise stretching the lower back and tightening the abdominal muscles. Keep your back straight. Repeat 10 times and anti-clockwise 10 times. This opens up the birth canal and prepares you for labour and birth.

3. Sit upright with arms out, breathing in lift the right leg in line with your hip, keeping the leg straight, balance and breathe out lowering the leg, repeat 10 times both legs. This helps the body maintain balance.

4. In cat curl position while using the ball to rest your head and chest on, let your arms hang loose. Breathe in and curl

your back (as in cat curl) up to the ceiling, pause, breathe out and relax.

IMPORTANT!

Take care not to hollow your back: it should always return to a straight/neutral position.

4.and 5. Relaxation and Connection

During your pregnancy, you will notice that you feel tired at times and if you do not relax enough you will notice this is more of an exhausted state, even when you have not been exerting yourself.

This is your body telling you that it needs that relaxed state to grow your Baby and keep you healthy.

If you have practiced yoga, use the relaxation and breathing techniques as often as you can. Even if you only do this for a few minutes every day, I promise, it will really help.

If you have never done yoga, take time to just sit, breathe and relax. Again, even if just for a few minutes every day.

If you don't your body will eventually make you one way or another, there is no doubt about that.

This is how complications occur, when you do not listen!

Myths exploded

Chapter 7

Myths exploded

1 My roots will show for 9 months!

Relax, minimal amounts of chemicals are absorbed through the skin when dyeing your hair.
If you are concerned use ammonia free products.

2 I cannot have my caffeine fix!

Chill, you can still enjoy your morning coffee.
Research has shown that that there is no clear link between caffeine and premature birth.
It's a good idea, however, not to overdo it whether pregnant or not.

3 Sushi is off limits!

Ask the Japanese, they know a thing or two about it, and they consider raw fish to be a good part of a pregnancy diet!
As long as the fish isn't high in mercury, it's considered safe.

4 You're grounded!

Enjoy, there is no reason that you cannot fly up to 37 weeks provided you have a certificate from your doctor or midwife to say that you and baby are healthy.

5 The cat has to go!

Kitty will do you more good than harm.
Cats are known to help relax us.
The hype about cleaning the litter trays is what has caused the concern.
The parasite that causes toxoplasmosis can live in the cat poo, however, so if you can avoid cleaning it, well why not?
If you can't, be sensible, wear gloves, wash hands thoroughly after cleaning and clean the box daily as the parasite becomes infectious between 1 and 5 days.
You are more likely to come into contact with this in the garden if you are working there and messing around with soil, so the same applies here! Leave the gardening to someone else.

6 Ditch the chocolate!

Reasons to eat chocolate: (Dark chocolate is best)
• Produces happy babies: - Research published in Finland suggests that pregnant women who ate chocolate gave birth to happy babies, more active and "positively reactive"
• Chocolate helps keep blood pressure stable.
• Chocolate contains copper, iron and magnesium.
• Chocolate relaxes you.
As with everything practice common sense and moderation.

7 No sex!

Lies! All lies! How did you get in this condition in the first place? As long as you and your Baby are healthy you can still enjoy sex.
You may find that you enjoy it more.... bonus!

8 I´m eating for two now!

Aw come-on, no one is buying that one.
Yes, you will need a few more calories perhaps by the time you get to around 28 weeks, but not for the whole pregnancy. Snacking can help if you feel nauseous, so eat some healthy

snacks, and a little bit of chocolate too!

9 The gym is out!

Hahaha...you can't get off that easy.

Exercise is good for you and the Baby.

There is no reason to change your exercise routine (if you have one) just listen to your body when it says enough!

You see it's ALL about FLOW!

All about U-turns

Chapter 8

All about U-turns

*I*f you watch television, surf the Net, read books (I hope so) or even talk to people it would appear that pregnancy is fraught with danger!

How can something that is a natural process engender so much fear?

It's not being pregnant that causes the fear it's all the "good" advice that comes with it.

Don't get me wrong it's all meant well, however, the damage that can be caused with the overload of rights and wrongs can far outweigh many of the "dangers."

Since the beginning of time there have been many theories and beliefs that after a time we have done a U-turn and "proved" them wrong.

So, what to believe?

- Your body was in the optimum condition to become pregnant.

- Whatever your lifestyle your body managed to balance all that was needed to achieve pregnancy.

Does that mean don't change anything?

Not necessarily, what it, means is:

- Use common sense
- Listen to your body
- Learn to connect to how you feel

If it doesn't feel right, or you feel unsure, don't do it, right now.

The more you can relax and enjoy your pregnancy, the happier and healthier your Baby is likely to be - as are you!

It's all about how you feel!
It's all about Flow!

Relax and take it easy.
You, Your Baby and your body have got this!

So, what next?

Chapter 9

So, what next?

*S*o, what next?

You have been Perfectly Pregnant for approximately 9 months / 40 weeks or thereabouts.

As we have seen, there is no such thing as exact timing; it will be near enough though.

Now your Baby's timer will start to ring.

Your body will begin giving you signals that Baby is now ready to come into the world.

In "Antenatal Care: Be Perfectly Pregnant...

A Simple and Empowering Guide to Pregnancy"

the follow-up to this book, we will look at:

- The changes in you and your Baby during pregnancy through the weeks
- How to prepare your mind and body.
- Nutrition.
- Exercise...and much more....

With this knowledge and practice, you will enjoy a unique experience and connection

Thank you

I would like to offer you a **FREE** gift of a "relaxation and connection recording for pregnancy", as a way of saying thanks for reading.

If you would like to receive this please send me an email to beperfectlypregnant@gmail.com subject "Free recording" and I will send you an mp3.

My promise to you:

I will not bombard you with unsolicited emails
I will not share your information with any third parties

Have a Healthy and Happy pregnancy.
Linda xc

Resources

Works Cited
Adler, Daphne. *Debunking the Bump: A Mathematician Mom Explodes Myths about Pregnancy*. S.l.: Daphne Adler Siniscalco, 2014. Print.

Dick-Read, Grantly. *Childbirth without Fear: The Principles and Practice of Natural Childbirth*. London: Pinter & Martin, 2013. Print.

Pinterest Boards:
https://uk.pinterest.com/linda9166/be-perfectly-pregnant/

If you want more information or would like to contact Linda :

Website: http://www.beperfectlypregnant.com

Facebook Page: https://www.facebook.com/lledwidge/

Email:beperfectlypregnant@gmail.com

NOTES

NOTES

20372603R00048

Printed in Poland
by Amazon Fulfillment
Poland Sp. z o.o., Wrocław